Hajer Nouira
Khouloud Rmili
Mohamed Fekih Hassen

SARS-Cov2-related dysthyroidism in intensive care patients

Hajer Nouira
Khouloud Rmili
Mohamed Fekih Hassen

SARS-Cov2-related dysthyroidism in intensive care patients

Incidence of dysthyroidism in intensive care patients with COVID-19 pneumonia and its prognostic impact

ScienciaScripts

Imprint

Cover image: www.ingimage.com

This book is a translation from the original published under ISBN 978-620-6-71947-2.

Publisher:
Sciencia Scripts
is a trademark of
Dodo Books Indian Ocean Ltd. and OmniScriptum S.R.L publishing group

120 High Road, East Finchley, London, N2 9ED, United Kingdom
Str. Armeneasca 28/1, office 1, Chisinau MD-2012, Republic of Moldova, Europe
Printed at: see last page
ISBN: 978-620-8-04448-0

SUMMARY E

INTRODUCTION

The neuroendocrine response plays an important role in the body's adaptation to acute and severe illness. This response is not merely an adaptive mechanism, but also a powerful means of defense aimed at preserving life and maintaining homeostatic equilibrium. This complex phenomenon orchestrates a cascade of significant hormonal responses, marking the onset of crucial metabolic and endocrine disturbances that could be mistaken for genuine endocrine diseases (1,2).

In December 2019, the world witnessed the appearance of a new coronavirus SARS-CoV-2 (Severe Acute Respiratory Syndrome CoronaVirus2) (3). Then, after a rapid and exponentially accelerating spread of cases worldwide, the World Health Organization (WHO) officially declared in March 2020 that it was a pandemic of major proportions, both in health and socio-economic terms (4).

As a cellular entry point, SARS-CoV-2 uses the angiotensin-converting enzyme type 2 (ACE2). The virus primarily targets the lung. Clinically, it is characterized by a high degree of inter-individual variability, ranging from a mildly symptomatic infection to severe pneumonia requiring oxygen therapy (in 14-29% of cases), or even to a critical form requiring transfer to the intensive care unit due to acute respiratory distress syndrome (ARDS), with a potentially fatal outcome. (5). However, in association with a cytokine storm, the range of associated disorders is very varied (5 to 12% of cases), including disruption of the endocrine system (6,7).

Thyroid dysfunction was one of the metabolic disorders sought and observed in COVID 19 patients.

The international scientific community has.responded.enormously.to. the.COVID-19.pandemic.and.has.carried.out.extensive.research.into.various.aspects.of.the. disease, including prevention, diagnosis and treatment. These studies have shown that dysthyroidism associated with COVID-19 infection is increasingly prevalent in intensive care settings (8). However, this entity was imperfectly described. To this end, we carried out a 2-year prospective study in the intensive care unit of the CHU Tahar Sfar de Mahdia, with the aim of :

- Determining the incidence of thyroid dysfunction in patients with SARS-CoV-2 pneumonia
- Assessing its prognostic impact

MATERIALS AND METHODS

1. TYPE, LOCATION AND PERIOD OF STUDY

This is a prospective monocentric study carried out in the Medical Intensive Care Unit at the 14-bed EPS Tahar Sfar in Mahdia. The study period was between September 01, 2020 and August 31, 2022.

2. STUDY PATIENTS

2.1. Inclusion criteria

All patients with the following criteria were included:

- Age over 18
- Hospitalized in the Medical Intensive Care Unit for pneumonia caused by
  SARS-CoV-2 and having a thyroid work-up on admission. Infection with this virus was confirmed by reverse transcription polymerase chain reaction (RT-PCR).

2.2 Exclusion criteria

We have excluded :

- Patients with previously diagnosed central or peripheral or autoimmune dysthyroidism
- Patients with a stay in another intensive care unit of more than 72 hours
- Care limitations

3. PROTOCOL AND METHOD

- All patients with the inclusion criteria had a 3cc venous sampling within the first 24 hours of hospitalization.
- Thyroid function tests included thyroid stimulating hormone (TSH) and free thyroxine (FT4) determinations. These assays were

performed by chemiluminescence on a Bechman Coulter Unicel Dxi 600.

4. DATA COLLECTION

- ❖ The data were collected prospectively on specific forms (designed for this work).
- ❖ From these files, we collected epidemiological, clinical, paraclinical, evolutionary and therapeutic data on all patients.

4.1. Anamnestic data

- ❖ Gender: masculine or feminine
- ❖ Age
- ❖ Comorbidities: hypertension, diabetes, dyslipidemia, asthma, chronic obstructive pulmonary disease (COPD), stroke, chronic renal failure (CRF), pregnancy.
- ❖ Background treatment
- ❖ Vaccination status covid-19
- ❖ Duration of symptoms before hospitalization
- ❖ Reason for admission to intensive care

4.2. Severity scores

- ❖ **The "APACHE II" score** (Acute Physiology And Chronic Health Evaluation II), in 1985(9)was based on 12 physiological variables making up the Acute Physiology Score (APS), to which age and certain pre-existing diseases were added. Each physiological variable is assessed during the first 24 hours of hospitalization in the intensive care unit, and scored on a scale ranging from 0 (normal range) to 4 (most abnormal value).
- ❖ **SAPS II" score** (10) (Simplified Acute Physiology Score II) was designed to measure the severity of illness in patients admitted to

intensive care units aged 18 and over. The score ranges from 0 to 163 points (taking into account the most pejorative values during the first 48 hours of hospitalization), while predicted mortality varies from 0 to 100%.

- **SOFA" score** (11) "Sequential sepsis-related Organ Failure assessment" is designed to assess sepsis-related organ dysfunction on the day of admission.

  It assesses 6 types of failure: neurological: assessment of Glasgow Coma Score (GCS); respiratory: calculation of PaO /FiO_{22} ratio; hemodynamic: assessment of mean arterial pressure and use of vasoactive drugs; hematological: platelet count; hepatic: bilirubin level; renal function: creatinemia according to age. The SOFA score ranges from 0 to 24 points.

4.3. Clinical parameters

- Clinical examination: (on day of admission to intensive care unit)
  - General signs: fever (temperature >38.3°C) or hypothermia (temperature ≤ 36°C).
  - Respiratory signs: respiratory frequency, signs of struggle ...
  - Neurological signs: state of consciousness was assessed by GCS.
  - Hemodynamic parameters: heart rate (HR), systolic blood pressure (SBP), diastolic blood pressure (DBP)

4.4. Paraclinical parameters

4.4.1. Biology

- Blood count (CBC); [leukocytes, lymphocytes and platelets], haemostasis work-up; prothrombin rate (PT), renal work-up (urea, creatinemia), blood ionogram (natremia, kalemia), liver work-up: aspartate aminotransferase (ASAT), alanine aminotransferase

(ALAT), arterial blood gas and inflammation marker: C-reactive protein (CRP).

- ❖ The tests were carried out in accordance with the usual methods used by the Biology Department at Tahar Sfar Hospital.

Definitions

- ❖ As defined by BERLIN (12)ARDS is diagnosed when the following four criteria are met:
  - ➢ Respiratory distress that began less than a week ago
  - ➢ Chest X-ray or CT scan showing bilateral lung opacities not explained by effusion, atelectasis or nodules
  - ➢ Respiratory failure not fully explained by cardiac failure or volume overload
  - ➢ Hypoxemia with a PaO2/FiO2 ratio < 300 mm Hg

Three stages of ARDS are defined:

- ✓ Mild ARDS: PaO2/FiO2 between 201 and 300 mm Hg with PEEP or CPAP ≥ 5 cm H2O
- ✓ ARDS moderate : PaO2/FiO2 ≤200 mm Hg with PEEP ≥ 5 cm H2O
- ✓ Severe ARDS: PaO2/FiO2 ≤ 100 mm Hg with PEEP ≥ 5 cm H2O.

- ❖ According to the French Society of Endocrinology, the various alterations in thyroid balance are defined as follows:
  - ➢ **Frustrated hypothyroidism** or **subclinical hypothyroidism**: TSH is low (usually between 4 and 10 mIU/L) and FT4 is normal (between 7.8 and 14.8pmol/L).

- **Primary hypothyroidism** or **peripheral hypothyroidism:** TSH is higher (> 10 mIU/L) and FT4 is low (< 7.8 pmol/L)
- **Central hypothyroidism**, **secondary hypothyroidism** or **thyrotropic insufficiency**: the diagnosis of hypothalamic-pituitary damage is based on the TSH/FT4 assay:
  - ✓ FT4 is consistently below the low threshold of normality.
  - ✓ TSH is not adapted to FT4 levels:
    - Low or normal levels indicate pituitary origin.
    - Slightly elevated, but still below 10-12 mIU/l, contrasting with a markedly low FT4. This biological representation suggests damage to the hypothalamus.
- **Peripheral hyperthyroidism** or **primary hyperthyroidism**: TSH levels are low (<0.3 mIU/L), while FT4 levels are high (>14.8 pmol/L).
- **Frustrated hyperthyroidism** or **subclinical hyperthyroidism**: TSH levels are low (<0.3 mIU/L), while FT4 is normal or at the upper limit of normal (between 7.8 and 14.8pmol/L).
- **Central hyperthyroidism:** TSH is normal (0.3 - 5.6 mIU/L) or slightly elevated, inappropriate for thyroid hyperhormonemia (> 14.8 pmol/L).

❖ according to K-DIGO 2012 (13) (*Kidney Disease: Improving Global Outcome)*, two parameters are taken into account to establish the diagnosis of acute renal failure (ARF) and its classification into stages of severity: elevation of creatininemia and volume of diuresis (Table I).

During an acute period, it is impossible to estimate glomerular filtration rate using the usual calculation methods MDRD, CKD-EPI...

Table I: Definition of ARF according to K-DIGO 2012

ARI stages	Creatininemia	Diuresis
1	Increase >26 µmol/l in 48 h **Or** >50% in 7 days	< 0.5 ml/kg/h for 6 to 12 h
2	Creatinine x 2 in 7 days	< 0.5 ml/kg/h during > 12h
3	Creatininemia x 3 in 7 days **Or** Creatinine >354 µmol/l (40 mg/L) in absence of previous value **Or** need to start dialysis	< 0.3 ml/kg/h >24h **Or** Anuria > 12 h

AKI: acute kidney injury **K-DIGO 2012:** Kidney Disease: Improving Global Outcome

4.4.2. Computed tomography (CT)

Computed tomography plays a key role in the initial diagnosis of COVID-19 and in assessing the extent of lung involvement.

The following radiological signs were described as compatible with COVID-19 pneumonia: ground-glass opacities, bilateral lesion involvement, peripheral distribution, multi-lobar involvement, posterior lesion topography, parenchymal condensations, crazy paving appearance (14).

Parenchymal damage is classified into 5 classes according to the percentage of lung affected: class 1 (absent or minimal damage < 10%), class 2 (moderate damage 10-25%), class 3 (significant damage 25-50%), class 4 (severe damage 50-75%) and class 5 (critical damage > 75%). (15).

4.5. Therapeutic and evolutionary parameters

- We also collected data on treatments administered throughout the ICU stay (corticosteroid therapy, anticoagulation and antibiotic therapy).
- We have followed the progress of all patients while specifying:

- Acute failures and/or complications: failure or success of high-flow oxygen (HFO), recourse to mechanical ventilation (MV), onset of septic shock or healthcare-associated infection.
- Length of stay in intensive care
- Duration of invasive mechanical ventilation
- Final outcome in intensive care :
  - ✓ Favourable: recovery with discharge home or transfer to another department
  - ✓ Death: cause of death

5. DATA ANALYSIS METHOD

Data were entered and analyzed using SPSS version 23 software.

5.1. Descriptive study

In the present study, qualitative variables are described in terms of numbers and percentages. Once normality has been verified, quantitative variables are expressed in terms of arithmetic mean (standard deviation), mode, median and interquartile range (IQR).

5.2. Analytical study

5.2.1. Varied Uni analytical study

The comparative study between two categorical variables was carried out using the Chi-square test or the Fischer test (if the size of one of the four cells is < 5).

For quantitative variables, Student's t-test or Mann-Whitney test were used, depending on the type of variable distribution.

5.2.2. Multi-variety analytical study

A multivariate analytical study using binary logistic regression was carried out, including parameters for which univariate analysis showed a p<0.2, in order to investigate factors associated with thyroid balance disturbance.

The significance level was set at 0.05.

6. ETHICAL CONSIDERATIONS

Ethical considerations were respected, namely anonymity and respect for patient confidentiality.

RESULTS

1. DESCRIPTIVE STUDY OF THE GENERAL POPULATION

During the study period, 449 patients were hospitalized. We excluded 85 patients. Reasons for exclusion were: previously diagnosed central or peripheral dysthyroidism or autoimmune disease, a stay in another intensive care unit of more than 72 hours, and limitations of care.

A total of 364 patients were included in our study. **Figure 1** illustrates the patient flow.

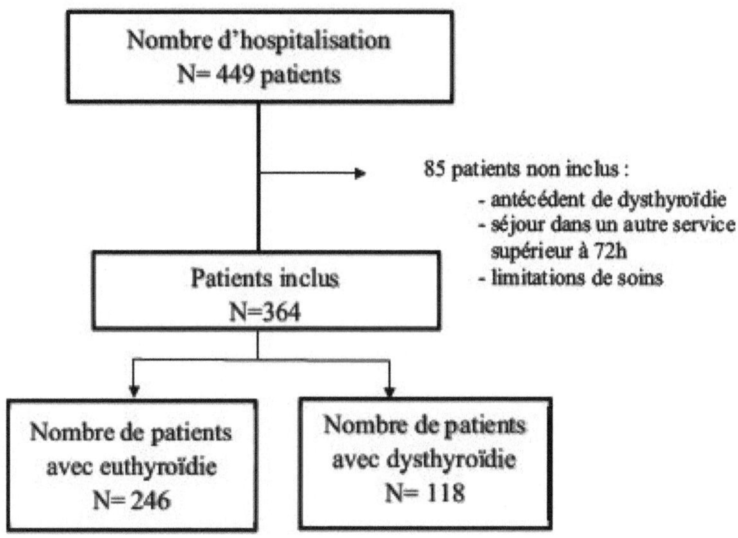

Figure 1: Flow chart for patients

1.1. Age

- The median age of patients was 61 years IQR [51-68].
- The most represented age group was 60-69 with 34.9%, followed by 50-59 with 21.7% (**Figure 2**).

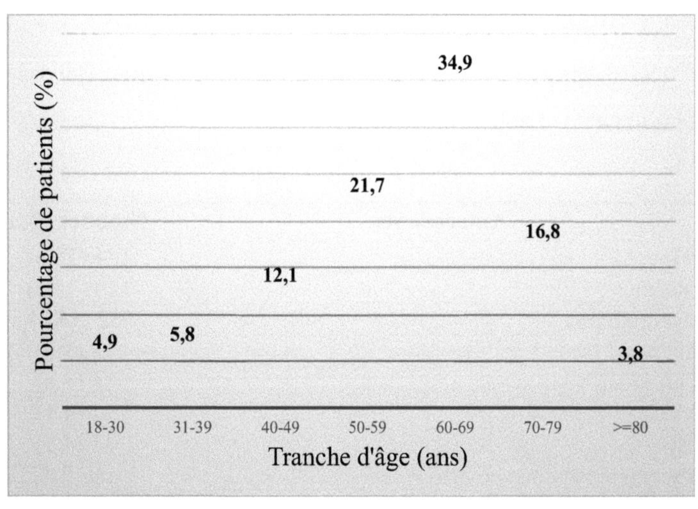

Figure 2: Patient distribution by age group (years)

1.2. Gender

Patients were predominantly male (207 men (56.9%)), with a sex ratio (M/F) equal to 1.32 (**Figure n°3**).

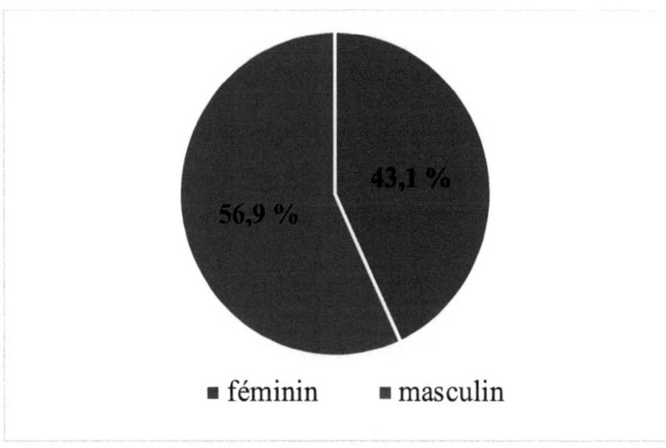

Figure 3: Distribution of patients by gender

1.3. History

The most frequent comorbidities were hypertension (39.6%) and diabetes (35.4%) (**Table II**).

Table II: Patient history

Antecedents	Number (%)
HTA	144 (39,6)
Diabetes	129 (35,4)
Dyslipidemia	52 (14,3)
Asthma	13 (3,6)
COPD	16 (4,4)
AVC	15 (4,1)
IRC	15 (4,1)
Vaccinated against covid-19	44(12,1)
Pregnancy	10 (2,7)

HTA: high blood pressure; COPD: chronic obstructive pulmonary disease
Stroke: cerebrovascular accident; CKD: chronic renal failure

1.4. Background treatment

In 6.8% of patients, long-term corticosteroids (oral and inhaled) are used as background treatment.

Antihypertensives (ACE inhibitors and angiotensin II receptor blockers) were used as background therapy in 22% of patients (**Table III**).

Table III: Use of corticoids and antihypertensives as background treatment

Background treatment	Number (%
Inhaled corticosteroid therapy	18 (4,9)
Oral corticosteroid therapy	7 (1,9)
IEC/ARA2	71 (22)

ACE inhibitors= Enzyme converting enzyme inhibitors;
ARA2= angiotensin II receptor antagonists

1.5. Previous home treatment

1.5.1. Home oxygenation

Of the patients, 45 or 12.4% were on oxygen therapy (by goggles or high-concentration masks) with a mean flow rate of 4.8 ± 2.3 L/min, and the median duration of oxygenation was 4 IQR days [2.25-6.75].

1.5.2. Corticosteroid therapy at home

Corticosteroid therapy was administered in 18 patients (4.9%), 12 of whom had dexamethasone injection with doses ranging from 6 to 8 mg/d. The average duration of corticosteroid use was 4 ±2 days.

1.6. Clinical profile

1.6.1. Reasons for admission to intensive care

Respiratory distress was the reason for admission in all patients.

1.6.2. Input mode

The majority of admissions came from emergency departments (75.5%), other hospital departments (17.3%) and other hospitals (7.1%).

1.6.3. The SAPS II score

On admission, median SAPS II was 26 IQR points [19-33] (Figure n°4).

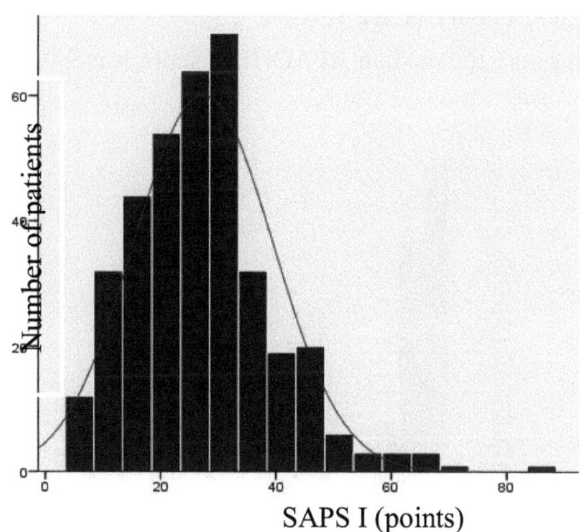

Figure 4: Distribution of patients by SAPS II score on admission

1.6.4. SOFA score

On admission to intensive care, the median SOFA score was 4 IQR points [3-4] (**Figure n°5**).

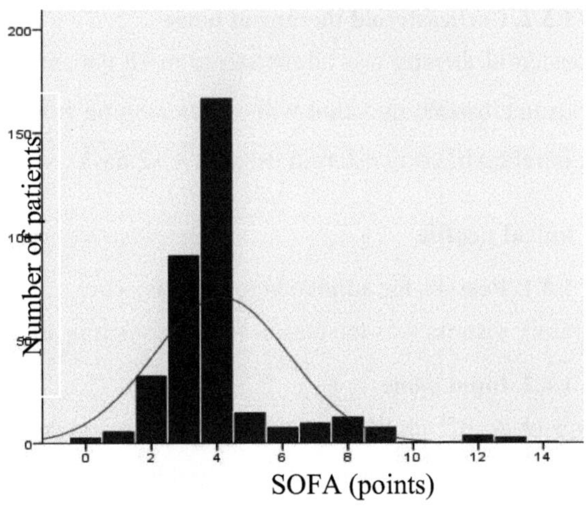

Figure 5: Distribution of patients by SOFA score on admission

1.6.5. The APACHE II score

On admission, the median APACHE II score was 9 IQR points [6-13] (Figure n°6).

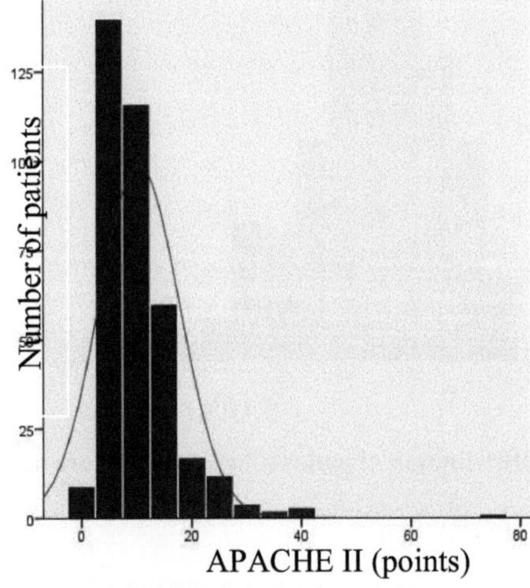

Figure 6: Distribution of patients by APACHE II score on admission

1.6.6. Duration of symptoms before hospitalization

The duration of symptom evolution before hospitalization was 7 IQR days [4-10].

1.6.7. Functional signs

Initial symptomatology was highly variable (Table IV).

1.6.7.1. Respiratory signs

Respiratory symptoms were dominated by dyspnoea in 91% of cases, followed by cough in 60%.

1.6.7.2. Digestive signs

Digestive symptoms included diarrhea in 7% of cases and vomiting in 5%.

1.6.7.3. Neurosensory symptomatology

Neurosensory symptomatology was presented by headaches in 15% of cases.

1.6.7.4. General signs

Fever was present in 52% of cases.

Table IV: Distribution of functional signs in symptomatic patients

The symptoms	Number (%)
Dyspnea	328 (91)
Cough	218 (60)
Chest pain	16 (4)
Rhinorrhea	9 (3)
Odynophagia	6 (2)
Diarrhea	26 (7)
Vomiting	17 (5)
Abdominal pain	13 (4)
Headaches	54 (15)
Anosmia	8 (2)
Agueusia	7 (2)
Other neurological disorders	13 (4)
Fever	186 (52)
Asthenia	183 (51)
Arthralgia-myalgia	59 (16)

1.7 Clinical examination

1.7.1. Entrance examination

On admission, 24 patients (6.6%) were in shock (**Table II**).

Table V: Patient examination on admission

	Number (%)
Fever	35 (9,6)
EDC	24 (6,6)
Coma	39 (11)

EDC: state of shock

1.7.2. Clinical forms

The majority of patients had severe ARDS (54% of cases), while 6 patients did not develop ARDS (**Table VI**).

Table VI: Distribution of patients according to Berlin classification

ARDS	Number (%)
Mild ARDS	28 (7,7)
Moderate ARDS	137 (37,6)
Severe ARDS	193 (53)
No ARDS	6 (1,7)

ARDS= Acute Respiratory Distress Syndrome

1.8. Paraclinical profile

1.8.1. Electrocardiogram

Seven patients (1.9%) with atrial fibrillation complete tachyarrhythmia (AFCT).

1.8.2. Radiology

In this study, chest CT scans were performed on 254 patients (69.8%). Lung involvement was predominantly severe or significant, in 38.9% and 33% of cases respectively.

Figure 7 illustrates the extent of lesions found on CT.

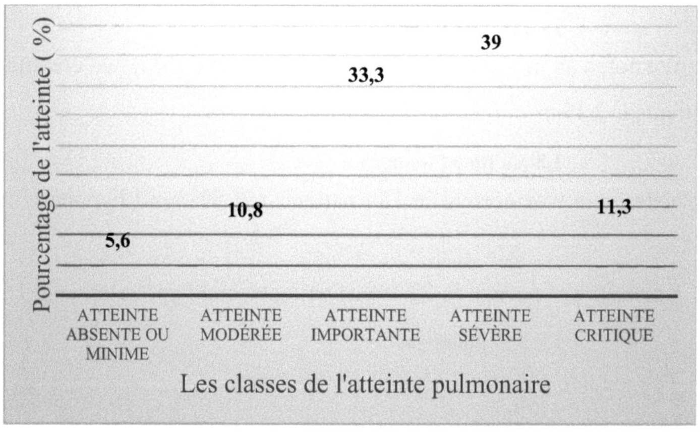

Figure 7: Extent of lung lesions on CT scan

1.8.3. Biology

1.8.3.1. Blood count

White blood cell count was normal in 52.2%.

One hundred and sixty-six patients (45.6%) had hyperleukocytosis and 8 patients (2.2%) had leukopenia (**Table VII**).

Lymphopenia was observed in 332 patients (91.2%).

Platelet count was within normal values in 75.8% of cases, thrombocytopenia was present in 32 patients (8.8%) and 56 patients (15.4%) had thrombocytosis.

1.8.3.2. Haemostasis work-up

TP was low in 65 patients (17.9%).

1.8.3.3. Marker of inflammation

CRP was above 6 mg/L in 360 patients (98.9%), with a median of 114 mg/L [68.25-170].

1.8.3.4. Liver function tests

AST and ALT levels were increased in 167 patients (45.9%) and 157 patients (43.1%) respectively.

1.8.3.5. Renal function

We noted an increase in urea in 173 patients (47.5%) and creatinine in 44 patients (12.1%).

1.8.3.6 Blood ionogram

Natraemia was normal in 189 patients (51.9%) and hyponatremia in 44.2%.

Kalemia was normal in 82.1% of patients, and hypokalemia in 16.8%.

1.8.3.7. Blood gas

- The median pH was 7.43 IQR [7.39- 7.46].
- Median PaCO2 was 36 mm Hg IQR [32- 41].
- The median PaO2/FiO2 ratio was 97 IQR [74- 142].

Table VII: Biological data on admission to the intensive care unit

Biological variables			
White blood cells (elements/mm³)	Median/IQR	*10580*	[7500-15030]
Lymphocytes (elements/mm³)	Median/IQR	800	[600- 1047]
Inserts (elements/mm³)	Average/standard deviation	292760	± 115381
TP (%)	Median/IQR	91%	[75-100]
CRP (mg/L)	Median/IQR	114	[68,25-170]
AST (UI/L)	Median/IQR	34	[24-53]
ALAT (UI/L)	Median/IQR	32	[20-52]
Urea (mmol/L)	Median/IQR	7,1	[5,125-10]
Creatinine (µmol/L)	Median/IQR	63	[51-81]
Natremia (mmol/L)	Median/IQR	136	[133-139]
Kalemia (mmol/L)	Median/IQR	4	[3,7-4,37]
pH	Median/IQR	7,43	[7,39-7,46]
PaO2 (mm Hg)	Median/IQR	77	[66-94]
PaCO2 (mm Hg)	Median/IQR	36	[32-41]
$HCO3^-$ (mmol/L)	Median/IQR	24	[21-26,7]
sO_2 (%)	Median/IQR	96	[93-98]
Lactates (mmol/L)	Median/IQR	2	[1,5-2,6]

TP: Prothrombin rate; CRP: C-reactive protein; ALAT: Alanine aminotransferase; ASAT: Aspartate aminotransferase; pH: hydrogen potential; PaO2: Oxygen partial pressure; PaCO2: Carbon dioxide partial pressure; $HCO3^-$: Bicarbonate; sO2: Oxygen saturation.

1.8.3.8. Thyroid work-up

In our study, 118 (32.4%) patients presented with thyroid disturbances. Hyperthyroidism was found in 105 cases (89%), while hypothyroidism was reported in 13 cases (11%).

Figure 8 illustrates the classification of identified thyroid disorders.

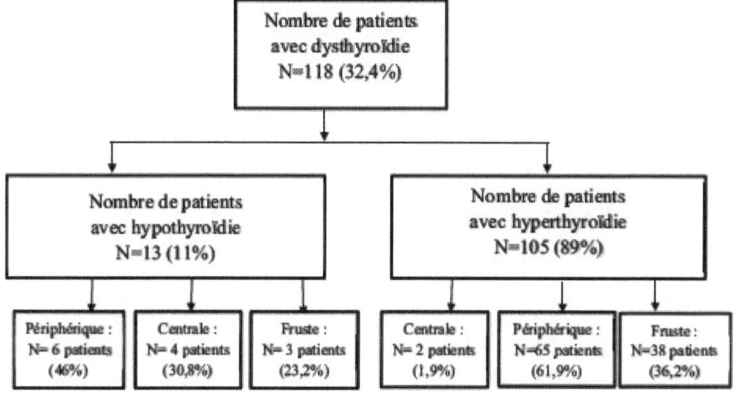

Figure 1Classification of thyroid disorders

1.9. Therapeutic profile

- ❖ The most commonly used oxygen therapy was OHD (73.1% of cases).
- ❖ Prone positions were used in 65.7% of cases.
- ❖ Anticoagulation was prescribed in all but 7 patients, and was divided according to dose into curative and preventive anticoagulation.
- ❖ Anticoagulation was preventive in 71.4% of cases and curative in 28.6% (**Table VIII**) .

Table VIII: Treatment of covid-19 patients in the ICU

The treatment	Number (%)
OHD	266 (73,1)
NIV	78 (21,4)
VMI	47 (12,9)

Average duration (days)	11 ± 6 days
DV	239 (65,7)
Dexamethasone	290 (79,7)
Anticoagulation :	
• preventive	255 (71,4)
• curative	102 (28,6)
Antibiotic therapy	78 (21,4)

OHD= high flow oxygen

NIV=non-invasive ventilation; IMV=invasive mechanical ventilation

DV= prone position

Evolution:

During their stay in the intensive care unit, 131 patients (41.3%) were secondarily intubated. Of these, 120 patients (91.6%) were curarized to optimize ventilation, with a median duration of mechanical ventilation of 9 IQR days [3-15].

1.10. Complications

1.10.1. Infectious complications

One hundred and sixty-three patients developed a nosocomial infection, complicating septic shock in 113 (31%).

The types of nosocomial infections are shown in **figure 9**:

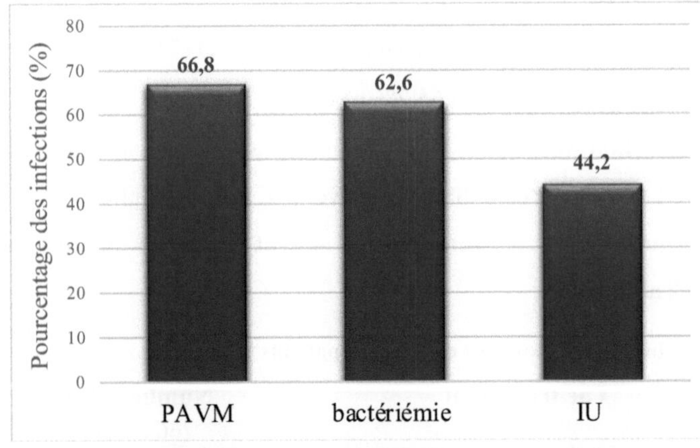

AVLP: Ventilator-associated lung disease; UTI: urinary tract infection

Figure 9: Healthcare-associated infections

1.10.2. Barotrauma complications

Pneumothorax occurred in 29 patients (8%), and 13 patients (3.6%) developed pneumomediastinum.

1.10.3. Thromboembolic complications

Pulmonary embolism (PE) was diagnosed in 10 patients (2.7%).

Six patients developed thrombophlebitis, and one patient suffered a stroke while hospitalized in intensive care.

1.10.4. Metabolic complications

Renal failure was observed in 82 patients (22.5%), of whom 28 (34.1%) underwent hemodialysis.

1.11. Length of stay

Median length of stay was 11 IQR days [5.25- 18].

1.12. Issue

In our study, mortality was 42.3%. The main causes of death were refractory hypoxemia (53.9%) and refractory shock (34.9%) (Figure 10).

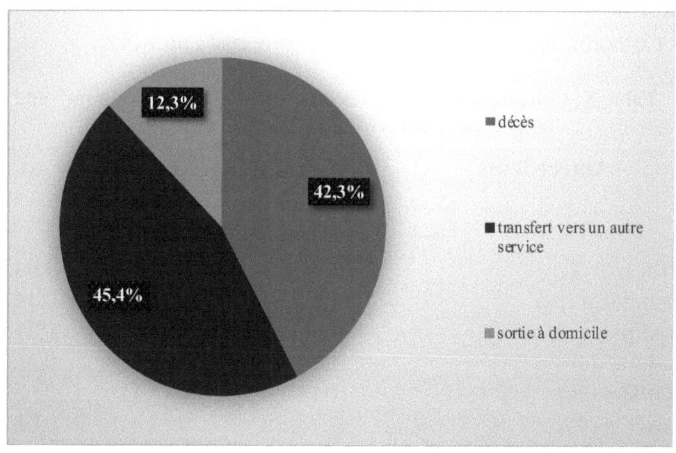

Figure 10: Patient outcomes

2. ANALYTICAL STUDY

2.1. The prognostic impact of dysthyroidism associated with COVID-19 infection

2.1.1. Univariate analytical study

2.1.1.1. Age and gender

No significant difference was found between the "Dysthyroidism" and "Euthyroidism" groups (**Table IX**).

Table IX: Comparison of age and gender between the two groups "Dysthyroidism" and "Euthyroidism".

	Euthyroidism N= 246	**Dysthyroidism N= 118**	**p**
Age (years) Median/IQR	61 [51-68]	59,5 [49-67,25]	0,326
Male n, (%)	137 (55,7)	70 (59,3)	0,513

2.1.1.2. History

Comorbidities were similar in both groups (**Table X**).

Table X: Comparison of histories between the "Dysthyroidism" and "Euthyroidism" groups

Antecedents	**Euthyroidism N= 246**	**Dysthyroidism N= 118**	**p**
HTA n (%)	97 (39,4)	47 (39,8%)	0,942
Diabetes n (%)	81 (32,9)	48 (40,7%)	0,148
Dyslipidemia n (%)	34 (13,8)	18 (15,3)	0,715
Asthma n (%)	10 (4,1)	3 (2,5%)	0,560
COPD n (%)	10 (4,1)	6 (5,1)	0,657
Stroke n (%)	11 (4,5)	4 (3,4)	0,782

CRI n (%)	9 (3,7)	6 (5,1)	0,576
Vaccinated against covid-19 n (%)	27 (11)	17 (14,4)	0,347
Pregnancy n (%)	6 (2,4)	4 (3,4)	0,733

HTA= hypertension; COPD= chronic obstructive pulmonary disease
CVA=Cerebrovascular Accident; CKD=Chronic Renal Failure

2.1.1.3. Background treatment

There was no significant difference between the two groups in the use of corticosteroids or antihypertensives (**ACEI/ARB2**) (**Table XI**).

Table XI: Comparison of background treatment between the "Dysthyroidism" and "Euthyroidism" groups

Background treatment	Euthyroidism N= 246	Dysthyroidism N= 118	p
Inhaled corticosteroids n (%)	11 (4,5)	7 (6)	0,535
Oral corticosteroid therapy n (%)	5 (2)	2 (1,7)	0,986
IEC/ARA2 n (%)	51 (22,7)	20 (20,2)	0,621

ARA2 : Angiotensin II receptor antagonists; ACEI : Converting enzyme inhibitors

2.1.1.4. Previous home treatment

Oxygen therapy and the use of home corticosteroids in the two study groups revealed no significant differences (**Table XII**).

Table XII: Treatment prior to hospitalization

	Euthyroidism N= 246	Dysthyroidism N= 118	p
O2 at home n (%)	30 (12,2)	15 (12,7)	0,889
Corticosteroid therapy n (%)	11 (4,5)	7 (5,9)	0,574

2.1.1.5. Severity scores

- ❖ The SAPS II score was significantly higher in the group of patients with dysthyroidism: 29 IQR [20.75-39] vs. 24 IQR [18-32]; p=0 .004 **(Figure no. 11).**
- ❖ The SOFA score was significantly different between the two groups (**Table XIII**).

Table XIII: Comparison of admission severity scores in the two groups

Severity scores On admission	Euthyroidism N= 246	Dysthyroidism N= 118	p
SOFA Median/ [IQR]	4 [3-4]	4 [3-5]	0,005
SAPS II Median/ [IQR]	24 [18-32]	29 [20,75-39]	0,004
APACHE II Médiane/ [IQR]	9 [6-12]	10 [6-14]	0,103

SAPS II: Simplified Acute Physiology Score II; SOFA: Sequential sepsis-related Organ Failure assessment; APACHE II: Acute Physiology And Chronic Health Evaluation II

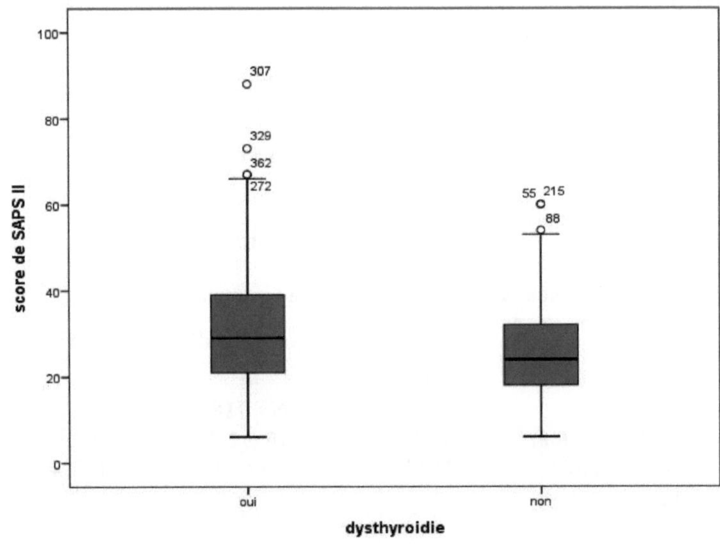

Figure 11: Comparison of the SAPS II score between the "Euthyroidism" and "Dysthyroidism" groups

2.1.1.6. Duration of symptoms before hospitalization

Duration was comparable in both groups (**Table XIV**).

Table XIV: Comparison of duration of symptoms before hospitalization between the two groups

	Euthyroidism N= 246	Dysthyroidism N= 118	p
Duration (days) Median/IQR	7 [4-10]	7 [4-10]	0,172

2.1.1.7. Functional signs

There were no significant differences in functional signs between the two groups (**Table XV**).

Table XV: Distribution of functional signs in the two groups

The symptoms	Euthyroidism N= 246	Dysthyroidism N= 118	p
Cough n (%)	143(58,6)	75(64,1)	0,318
Dyspnea n (%)	219(89,8)	109(93,2)	0,293
Chest pain n (%)	12(4,9)	4(3,4)	0,517
Rhinorrhea n (%)	8(3,3)	1(0,9)	0,281
Odynophagy n (%)	4(1,6)	2(1,7)	0,986
Diarrhea n (%)	18(7,4)	8(6,8)	0,853
Vomiting n (%)	14(5,7)	3(2,6)	0,183
Abdominal pain n (%)	10(4,1)	3(2,6)	0,560
Headache n (%)	39(16)	15(12,8)	0,430
Anosmia n (%)	6(2,5)	2(1,7)	0,910
Agueusia n (%)	6(2,5)	1(0,9)	0,435
Other neurological disorders n (%)	11(4,5)	2(1,7)	0,237
Fever n (%)	131(53,7)	55(47)	0,235
Asthenia n (%)	125(51,2)	58(49,6)	0,768
Arthralgia-myalgia n (%)	40(16,4)	19(16,2)	0,970

2.1.1.8. Clinical examination

No significant differences were found between the two groups (**Table XVI**) .

Table XVI: Comparison of clinical parameters between the two groups

Parameters	Euthyroidism N= 246	Dysthyroidism N= 118	p
Temperature (°C) Median/IQR	37 [37-37,6]	37 [36,77-38]	0,456
HR (bpm) Average/standard deviation	87,26 ± 19,08	91,58 ± 21,58	0,063
PAS (mm Hg) Median/IQR	130 [120-140]	130 [120-140]	0,714
PAD (mm Hg) Median/IQR	70 [70-80]	70 [60-80]	0,175
EDC n (%)	11(4,5)	13(11,1)	0,17

HR= heart rate; SBP= systolic blood pressure
DBP= diastolic blood pressure; DSC= state of shock

2.1.1.9. Acute respiratory distress syndrome

Forms of ARDS were similar between the two groups (Table XVII).

Table XVII: Comparison of ARDS forms in the two groups

ARDS	Euthyroidism N= 246	Dysthyroidism N= 118	p
ARDS Mild n (%)	20 (8,1)	8 (6,7)	0,98
Moderate ARDS n (%)	97 (39,4)	40 (33,9)	0,9
Severe ARDS n (%)	124 (50,4)	69 (58,5)	0,15
No ARDS n (%)	5 (2,1)	1 (0,9)	0,053

ARDS: acute respiratory distress syndrome

2.1.1.10. Thoracic CT scan

The extent of lung lesions on CT was similar between the two groups (**Table XVIII**) .

Table XVIII: Comparison of CT lung involvement between the two groups

Classes of pulmonary involvement	Euthyroidism N= 170	Dysthyroidism N= 84	p
Minimal damage n (%)	8 (72,7)	3 (27,3)	0,676
Moderate disease n (%)	13 (61,9)	8 (38,1)	0,609
Significant damage n (%)	44 (67,7)	21 (32,3)	0,879
Severe disease n (%)	51 (67,1)	25 (32,9)	0,969
Critical damage n (%)	15 (68,2)	7 (31,8)	0,896

2.1.1.11. Biology

- Median white blood cell count was significantly higher in the "Dysthyroidism" group; 11830 /mm³ [7700-16887.5] vs 9980 /mm³ [7497.5-13960]; p=0.025.
- The median lymphocyte count was significantly lower in the "Dysthyroidism" group; 735/mm³ [600-952.5] vs 800/mm³ [600-1100]; p=0.029 **(Table XIX)**.

Table XIX: Comparison of biological data on admission between the two groups

Biological variables	Euthyroidism N= 246	Dysthyroidism N= 118	p
White blood cells (elements/mm³) Median/IQR	*9980* [7497,5 - 13960]	11830 [7700 - 16887,5]	0,025
Lymphocytes (elements/mm³) Median/IQR	800 [600 - 1100]	735 [600 - 952,5]	0,029
Inserts (elements/mm³) Average/standard deviation	293313,01 ±115388,37	291610,17± 115850,63	0,895
TP (%) Median/IQR	93 [77,75 - 100]	85 [73 - 98]	0,008
CRP (mg/L) Median/IQR	110 [65 - 165,5]	119 [70 - 188]	0,235
AST (IU/L) Median/IQR	33 [24 - 49]	36,5 [24 - 64,75]	0,075

ALAT (IU/L) Median/IQR	*31,5* [19 - 50]	33[21,75-58,25]	0,357
Urea (mmol/L) Median/IQR	7 [5 - 9,17]	8 [5,9 - 11,1]	0,031
Creatinine (µmol/L) Median/IQR	61 [50 - 78]	67,5 [53 - 92,25]	0,066
Natremia (mmol/L) Median/IQR	136 [133 - 138,5]	137[134 - 139]	0,258
Kalemia (mmol/L) Median/IQR	4 [3,68 - 4,35]	4[3,74 - 4,38]	0,345
pH Median/IQR	7,43 [7,39 - 7,46]	7,42 [7,36 - 7,46]	0,082
PaO2 (mm Hg) Median/IQR	78 [68 - 94]	72 [64,75 - 95,25]	0,195
PaCO2 (mm Hg) Median/IQR	36 [32 - 40]	37 [32,75 - 43]	0,139
$HCO3^-$ (mmol/L) Median/IQR	24 [21,2 - 26,7]	24 [21 - 27]	0,469
sO_2 (%) Median/IQR	96 [94 - 98]	95 [91 - 97,25]	0,061
Lactates (mmol/L) Median/IQR	1.9 [1,4 - 2,5]	2,05 [1,57 - 2,6]	0,056

PT: Prothrombin rate; CRP: C-reactive protein; ALAT: Alanine aminotransferase ; ASAT: Aspartate aminotransferase; pH: hydrogen potential; PaO2: partial pressure of oxygen; PaCO2: Carbon dioxide partial pressure; $HCO3^-$: Bicarbonate; sO_2: Oxygen saturation

2.1.1.12. Intensive care treatment

2.1.1.12.1. Non-invasive respiratory assistance

- MHC use was comparable between the two groups; "Euthyroidism" (31.7%) vs. "Dysthyroidism" (33.9%); p=0.676.
- OHD was more widely used in the "Euthyroidism" group; 76.8% vs. 65.3% with a significant difference; p= 0.02.
- NIV use was comparable between the two groups (18.7% vs. 27.1%); p= 0.067 (**Table XX**).

2.1.1.12.2. Invasive respiratory assistance

The "Dysthyroidism" group required more VMI with a significant difference (19.5% vs. 9.8%; p = 0.01), with a comparable duration between the two groups; 10 IQR days [4 - 18] vs. 9 IQR days [5 - 15]; p= 0.847.

2.1.1.12.3. Ventral decubitus (VD)

The prone position was used more often in the "Dysthyroidism" group (67.8% vs. 64.6%), with no significant difference between the two groups; p=0.552.

Table XX: Comparison of ventilation modes between the two groups

Means of oxygenation	Euthyroidism N= 246	Dysthyroidism N= 118	p
MHC n (%)	78 (31,7)	40 (33,9)	0,676
OHD n (%)	189 (76,8)	77 (65,3)	0,02
NAV n (%)	46 (18,7)	32 (27,1)	0,067
VMI n (%)	24(9,8)	23(19,5)	0,01
Duration (days) Median/IQR	9 [5-15]	10 [4-18]	0,847
Curare n (%)	21 (91,3)	20 (90,9)	1
DV n (%)	159 (64,6)	80(67,8)	0,552

MHC= high concentration mask; OHD= high flow oxygen
NIV= non-invasive ventilation; IMV= invasive mechanical ventilation; VD= prone position

2.1.1.12.4. Corticosteroid therapy

- Dexamethasone was prescribed in 84.6% of patients with normal thyroid function versus 69.5% in the dysthyroid group; p=0.001.
- Methylprednisolone was used significantly more in the "Dysthyroidism" group; 57.6% vs. 43.9% with p= 0.014.

2.1.1.12.5. Anticoagulation

- No significant difference was found between the two groups studied with regard to the nature of anticoagulation (**Table XXI**) .

Table XXI: Comparison of the nature of anticoagulation between the two groups

Anticoagulation	Euthyroidism N= 243	Dysthyroidism N= 114	p
Curative n (%)	71 (29,2)	31 (27,2)	0,08
Preventive n (%)	172 (70,8)	83 (72,8)	

2.1.1.12.6. Antibiotic therapy

Antibiotic treatment was prescribed more frequently in the "Dysthyroidism" group (22.9%) versus 20.7% in the "Euthyroidism" group, although the difference was not significant (p=0.64).

2.1.1.12.7. Use of catecholamines

The introduction of vasoactive drugs was more frequent in the "Dysthyroidism" group (55.1% vs. 32.4%); $p < 10^{-3}$.

2.1.1.13. Length of stay

Length of stay in the intensive care unit was comparable between the two groups, with p= 0.33 (**Table XXII**).

Table XXII: Comparison of length of stay between the two groups

	Euthyroidism N= 246	**Dysthyroidism N= 118**	**p**
Length of stay in intensive care (days) Median/IQR	11 [5-17]	11 [6-20]	0,330

2.1.1.14. Complications

- The rate of nosocomial infections was significantly higher in the "Dysthyroidism" group: 67 patients (56.8%) vs. 96 patients (39%); p= 0,001.

  The same applies to septic shock; 55 (46.6%) vs 58 (23.6%); $p < 10^{-3}$.
- There was no significant difference between the two groups studied in terms of thromboembolic complications.
- The "Dysthyroidism" group developed ARF significantly more frequently during their ICU stays. Indeed, 30.5% of this group developed this complication, whereas it was only found in 18.7% of the "Euthyroidism" group (p=0.012).
- The main complications are shown in **Table XXIII**.

Table XXIII: Comparison of complications between the two groups

Complications	Euthyroidism N= 246	Dysthyroidism N= 118	p
Nosocomial infections n (%)	96 (39)	67 (56,8)	0,001
Septic EDC n (%)	58 (23,6)	55 (46,6)	< 10^{-3}
Pulmonary embolism n (%)	7 (2,8)	3 (2,5)	0,98
IRA n (%)	46(18,7)	36 (30,5)	0,012
Hypokalemia n (%)	17 (6,9)	14 (11,9)	0,113
Hyperkalemia n (%)	10 (4,1)	9 (7,6)	0,153
Hyponatremia n (%)	11 (4,5)	2 (1,7)	0,237
Hypernatremia n (%)	10 (4,1)	4 (3,4)	1
Cytolysis n (%)	6 (2,4)	4 (3,4)	0,733

ARF= *Acute* Renal Failure; SH= Shock

2.1.1.15. Rhythm disorder

TACFA was encountered less frequently in the "Dysthyroidism" group (5.1%) than in the "Euthyroidism" group (6.9%), although the difference was not significant; p= 0.503.

2.1.1.16. Mortality

The mortality rate was higher in the "Dysthyroidism" group with a statistically significant difference; 63 (53.4%) vs 90 (36.7%) with p= 0.003.

2.1.2. Multi-variety analytical study

In the multivariate analysis, corticosteroid therapy and preventive anticoagulation were factors independently associated with dysthyroidism (Table XXIV).

Table XXIV: Multivariate analysis of factors predictive of the occurrence of dysthyroidism associated with COVID-19 infection

Parameters	p	OR	95% CI
Corticosteroid therapy	0,045	*0,033*	0,001 - 0,932
Anticoagulation	0,013	*61,38*	2,422 - 1556,02

DISCUSSION

COVID-19 is a multi-systemic disease caused by infection with SARS-CoV-2. It is generally not very symptomatic, and respiratory disorders are the most serious aspect. It can be life-threatening, so covid-19-positive patients may present with mild symptoms or even severe hypoxic respiratory failure, with a marked alteration in the ventilation/perfusion ratio. (16).

Although considered a respiratory disease, other organs and systems can be affected by COVID-19, notably the thyroid. Indeed, the literature has highlighted the relationship established between COVID-19 and the various disturbances in thyroid balance since the outbreak of this pandemic. In this context, we sought to assess the association between COVID-19 and thyroid function, as well as the potential of thyroid hormones to predict the severity of COVID-19.

Following infection with SARS-CoV-2, thyroid disruption may result primarily from two mechanisms: direct invasion of the endocrine glands by the virus, and action exerted by inflammatory mediators and immune response cells (17).

For direct infection, the angiotensin-converting enzyme 2 (ACE2) plays an important role in the internalization of SARS-CoV-2 into host cells, thus contributing significantly to the pathogenesis of COVID-19. Indeed, the virus is equipped with a spike glycoprotein, also known as Spike protein or S protein, consisting of S1 and S2 subunits. When it binds to ACE2, the S1 subunit separates from the ACE2 receptor, a process that requires the presence of transmembrane serine protease 2 (TMPRSS2). This separation leads to a conformational change, facilitating membrane fusion and enabling the virus to enter host cells (18).

These receptors are widely expressed in several tissues, including thyroid follicular cells, as suggested by direct molecular analysis performed on surgical samples of thyroid tissue. This expression makes the thyroid gland susceptible to damage following infection with SARS-CoV-2. Virus intrusion and multiplication within these cells could cause direct cellular damage, possibly leading to programmed inflammatory cell death (19).

In addition to the direct impact on thyroid or pituitary cells, it is crucial to consider another potential process: the indirect repercussions of the inflammatory response triggered by COVID-19 infection and mediated by the immune system. Immune-mediated injury is triggered by a variety of cells and cytokines. Recently, the mechanisms of the immune response to COVID-19 have come under scrutiny, highlighting the importance of CD4+ and CD8+ T cells in the different targets of SARS-CoV-2. These cells play a crucial role in fighting the infection, and also persist into the resolution phase of the disease. In addition, an elevated number of T helper (Th) 17 cells and a reduced ratio of regulatory T cells to Th17 cells, combined with elevated serum interleukin (IL)-6 levels, could contribute to the disproportionate cytokine release frequently observed in individuals with severe disease. Various cytokines and chemokines, such as IL-1 beta, IL-2, IL-4, IL-6, IL-8, IL-17, IL-22, tumor necrosis factor alpha, interferon gamma, granulocyte colony-stimulating factor, IFN-gamma-induced protein 10 and monocyte chemoattractant protein 1, could also play a role in the development of COVID-19, particularly in its severe form.

These responses, both cellular and humoral, help trigger the severe inflammatory reaction known as the "cytokine storm", often associated with severe forms of disease and acute respiratory distress syndrome.

As a result of this pronounced imbalance in the immune system, patients with autoimmune thyroid disease could present a more severe clinical course of COVID-19 attributable to initially higher levels of serum IL-6 and TNF-alpha than healthy individuals. At the same time, SARS-CoV-2 could break down immunotolerance in predisposed patients, triggering a new manifestation of immune-mediated thyroiditis, aggravating pre-existing thyroid disease or inducing recurrence (20,21).

Thyroid disorders have also been reported following vaccination against SARS-CoV-2 (22). It should be noted that from the very start of COVID-19 vaccination campaigns, some studies have shown the emergence of thyroid disease, in particular thyroiditis. According to one systematic review, thyroid dysfunction occurs on average 11 days after vaccination (23). To explain the relationship between COVID-19 vaccination and thyroid disease, the first proposed mechanism is adjuvant-induced autoimmune/inflammatory syndrome (24,25).

However, it has been shown that antibodies to SARS-CoV-2 proteins can cross-react with tissue antigens, notably thyroid peroxidase (26). However, considering that billions of COVID-19 vaccines have already been administered worldwide, the appearance of dysthyroidism following vaccination is a very rare side effect (22).

The incidence of dysthyroidism in our study was 32.4%. Hyperthyroidism was found in 105 cases (89%), while hypothyroidism was detected in 13 cases (11%). Univariate analysis revealed that the group of patients with dysthyroidism was more severe: the SAPS II score was significantly higher. Similarly, use of mechanical ventilation, administration of catecholamines, rate of nosocomial infections and occurrence of septic DCI were significantly higher. Mortality was higher in the "Dysthyroidism" group (53.4% vs. 36.7%). In the multivariate analysis, corticosteroid therapy and preventive anticoagulation were factors independently associated with dysthyroidism.

In our study, the median age of patients was 61 years IQR [51-68]. According to the study by Oliveira et al (227)the study by Grasselli et al (228)and the study by Yu et al (29)the median age was 61 ±11 years, 63 ±7 years and 64 ±7 years respectively (**Table XXV**).

Table XXV: The age variation observed in individuals with COVID-19 according to various studies

Study	Country	Sample size	Average age
Grasselli et al [28]	Italy	3988	63 ±7
Oliveira et al [27]	United States	1283	61 ±11
Yu et al [29]	China	226	64 ±7
Our study	Tunisia	364	61[51-68]

Our study revealed a male predominance (56.9%) with a sex ratio of 1.32.The results presented in a study from the Avicenne military hospital in Marrakech (330) also revealed male predominance (91.8% vs. 8.2%) in a population of 318 patients, with an estimated sex ratio of 11. The study by Yu et al. (29) and Mutair et al (331) also showed a predominance of males, with a sex ratio of 1.59 and 8.09 respectively.

This male susceptibility was the subject of an Italian study by Federico et al. (332). The study focused on two parameters triggering COVID-19 infection; ACE2 and TMPRSS2, both of which are influenced by sex. Firstly, the gene coding for ACE2 is expressed on the X chromosome and is influenced by estrogen levels, explaining its high level in women. Its role is to ensure the proper functioning of the renin-angiotensin system (RAS) in all the systems concerned. Once viral infection has been proven, the RAS has a vasodilatory, anti-inflammatory and anti-fibrotic action. On the other hand, lower androgen levels in women help maintain a reduced level of TMPRSS2, representing an additional protective factor. Consequently, these mechanisms explain the role of hormones and sex chromosomes in men's vulnerability to SARS-CoV-2 infection (332).

Hypertension (39.6%), followed by diabetes (35.4%), were the most common comorbidities in our study. Indeed, hypertension was present in 55% and 42.5% respectively in the study by Donamou et al. (333) and Yu et al (29). Whereas in the study by Oliveira et al (27) and the study by Al Mutair et al (331)diabetes was present in 41.2% and 43.8% of cases respectively.

According to studies carried out in intensive care, mortality was over 50% in diabetic and hypertensive patients. In the study by Al Mutair et al. (331)mortality was 75% in diabetic patients and 81% in patients with hypertension. In the study by Grasseli et al (228)mortality was 63.8% for diabetics and 58.5% for hypertensives.

According to an Indian study published in 2020 (334) diabetes, in addition to its role in the occurrence of infection, favours the occurrence of four main phenomena which are thought to contribute to the pathophysiology of COVID-19 :

- Overexpression of ACE2
- Overexpression of furin, a membrane protease that facilitates
- intracellular entry of coronaviruses.
- Impaired T-cell function
- Increased Interleukin 6 levels

There were no specific clinical features to distinguish COVID-19 from other viral respiratory infections. However, a variety of clinical manifestations were observed, ranging from pauciously symptomatic forms to suggestive pneumonia (with or without signs of severity; ARDS, or even multi-visceral failure). However, forms with digestive symptoms, confusional state, initially non-febrile, are often prominent in the elderly, according to the study by Devaux et al. (335).

According to our study, the most frequently observed functional signs on admission were dyspnea (91%), cough (60%) and fever (52%).

Dyspnea was observed in 90.4% of cases in the study by Hariyanto et al. (336) and noted in 84.9% of cases in the study by Al Mutair et al. (331) at the time of admission.

Cough was observed in 71.1% of cases in the study by Xu et al. (337) and 81% in the study by Donamou et al. (333).

Fever was reported in 40.5% and 71.1% of cases respectively in the study by Oliveira et al.(227) in the study by Saha et al (338). It may be absent when the patient is admitted, but may develop during hospitalization as a result of taking antipyretics at home.

Tachycardia was found in 74% of cases in Donamou's study (333) et al, in 4% of cases in the study by Yu et al (29). Whereas in our study, tachycardia was present in 20.9% of cases.

It has been demonstrated that (39) that SOFA, APACHE II and SAPS II scores are predictive of mortality in COVID-19 patients.

Most intensive care studies found a median SOFA of between 4 and 6 at D1; the median SOFA was 6 in the studies by Raschke et al (440)Jiqian et al (441) and Mitra et al (442). In the study by Schmidt et al (443)the median was 5. A median of 4 was found in the studies by Yu et al. (29) and Xu et al (337). This result was confirmed in our series, where we found a median SOFA of 4 IQR points [3-4].

The most characteristic radiological abnormalities in COVID-19 pneumonia are multifocal, bilateral, asymmetric ground-glass areas (80% of cases). Involvement typically predominates in the peripheral, posterior and basal regions. Micronodular syndrome, excavation, septal lines and mediastinal adenomegaly are generally absent. (14,444).

In severe forms, lesions are more extensive and the proportion of pulmonary condensation is higher than that of ground glass (445).

According to Grillet et al, thoracic CT with contrast injection in suspected patients with a severe clinical condition or clinical suspicion of pulmonary embolism is necessary to rule out the diagnosis of pulmonary embolism, and to make the diagnosis in the event of negative PCR by showing typical scannographic images. (446).

In our study population, lymphopenia was found in 91.2% of cases, with a median of 800/mm3 IQR [600 - 1047]. This was the most common blood count abnormality observed in the various studies. Indeed, according to the study by Mitra et al. (442) and Jiqian et al (447)lymphopenia was observed in the majority of patients, with medians of 800/mm3 IQR [500-1000] and 600/mm3 IQR [500-800] respectively.

The study by Yu et al (29) found a median leukocyte count of 8540 /mm3 IQR [5890 - 12690] on admission. This was also the case in the study by Xu et al (337)with a median of 8300 /mm3 IQR [5600 - 10300]. Whereas in our study, a higher median was found at 10580/mm3 IQR [7500-15030].

Transaminases (AST and ALAT) were statistically higher in severe forms of COVID-19 (48,49). In our series, hepatic cytolysis was reported in 45.9% of cases (ASAT elevated) and 43.1% of cases (ALAT elevated). Whereas in Guan's study (550) the percentage was 21.3%. On the other hand, this result was close to 31% in the series by Zhou (551).

In our study series, hyperuremia was found in 47.5% and increased creatinemia in 12.1% of patients, with medians of 7.1 mmol/L IQR [5.125 - 10] and 63 µmol/ L IQR [51 - 81] respectively. In the study by Yu et al (30)study, urea and creatinine values increased significantly, with medians of 7.34 mmol/L IQR [5.2- 14.1] and 64.2 µmol/ L IQR [49 - 111.6] respectively.

In the literature, the marker of inflammation "CRP" was increased in most patients hospitalized in the ICU. A median CRP of 114 mg/L IQR [68.25 - 170] was reported in our series. This result was close to that reported in the study by Oliveira et al(28) which was 115 mg/L IQR [59 - 186.3].

Therapeutically, the percentage of patients requiring invasive mechanical ventilation differs from study to study: in our study, 49% of patients hospitalized with COVID-19 had IMV. In the study by Schmidt et al (443) and Biccard et al (552)the respective percentages of 63% and 40.1% of patients with mechanical ventilation were reported. Whereas in the study by Jiqian et al. (441)only 18% of patients required intubation.

Treatment recommendations vary from country to country, depending on the national protocol in place.

However, both the literature and the WHO agree that corticosteroids, in particular dexamethasone at a dose of 6 mg/d for 10 days, reduce ICU mortality, particularly in patients requiring oxygenation. (553).
Corticosteroids possess anti-inflammatory properties that could be useful in dysregulated systemic inflammation. The results of clinical studies strongly suggest that corticosteroid therapy may be effective in preventing clinical deterioration in patients with COVID-19. Specifically, a single daily dose of dexamethasone (6 mg) over 10 days reduced mortality at 28 days in patients requiring invasive mechanical ventilation (553). In addition, early inhalation of budesonide reduced the likelihood of urgent medical care and recovery time in patients with mild COVID-19 (554). It also reduced hospital admissions and deaths in symptomatic individuals at higher risk of complications (555). All these studies have highlighted the beneficial effect of adrenal steroids in improving the outcome of patients with COVID-19.
Although glucocorticoids play a protective role in the survival of some patients. Excessive cortisol production or prolonged corticosteroid treatment could increase mortality associated with COVID-19 through induction of immune deficiency, increased risk of opportunistic infections and development of hypothalamic-pituitary axis dysfunction (556). Prolonged or poorly controlled use has other serious side effects, including psychosis, hyperglycemia and the development of iatrogenic adrenal insufficiency (557) In particular, patients with severe forms who have received dexamethasone are at increased risk of adrenal insufficiency.

In addition to its beneficial effect in preventing thromboembolic complications, heparin has anti-inflammatory properties.

In fact, a systematic review concluded that heparin can reduce the concentration of inflammatory markers and improve patient health (58, 59). A meta-analysis revealed that adjunctive treatment with low-molecular-weight heparin can lower the risk of 7-day mortality by 48% and the risk of 28-day mortality by 37%, in particular to significantly improve the PaO2/FiO2 ratio (the improvement is particularly significant in the subgroup receiving high doses of LMWH ≥ 5000 units/day) (58,660). Heparin may therefore prove beneficial in patients with COVID-19. From a pathophysiological point of view, infection with covid-19 can lead directly or indirectly to dysfunction of the vascular endothelium, thereby increasing the risk of thrombosis. The virus enters endothelial cells primarily by binding to ACE-2. The study by Varga et al. showed the presence of viral elements in the endothelial cell and endothelial inflammation known as "endothelitis". Endothelial cell activation can have two main effects. The result is a well-coordinated innate immune response through the recruitment of immune cells, overexpression of chemotactic molecules and adhesion molecules, and activation of neutrophils, monocytes and platelets. In parallel, when the endothelium is dysfunctional and inflammatory, it will express tissue factor, which is the key to triggering the coagulation cascade. These two phenomena are designed to control infection and repair endothelial damage. However, they can become harmful if excessive and/or not controlled by the host, leading to widespread endothelial dysfunction. In addition, the induced cytokine storm, with its high release of interleukin-6, interleukin-8 and Tumor Necrosis Factor alpha, which also promote excessive tissue factor expression, activates extrinsic coagulation. Similarly, severe hypoxemia is a risk factor for pulmonary vasoconstriction and thromboembolic complications. Finally, it should be pointed out that some patients with

COVID-19 have developed anti-phospholipid antibodies and presented with strokes with obstruction of the limb arteries. This may be explained by the fact that anti-β2-glycoprotein I antibodies may also play a role in coagulopathy by causing an increase in pro-inflammatory mediators and adhesion molecules (661).

In our series, vasopressors were administered in 39.8% of cases. The study by Oliveira et al (227) showed a need for vasopressor drugs in 72.5% of cases, while in the study by Yu et al (29) and Donamou et al (333)only 21.2% and 9% of cases respectively. Hemodynamic failure is rare. It is often secondary to hypovolemia, cardiac damage or reventilation collapse.

Our study showed that the median length of hospital stay for intensive care patients was 11 IQR days [5.25- 18]. A study carried out in France during the first wave between March 1 and June 15, involving 90,800 patients, showed that the median length of hospital stay was 20 days when the patient had been in intensive care. This was reduced to 8 days if the patient had only undergone conventional hospitalization (662).

In our series, 22.5% of patients had developed functional renal failure. However, according to the cohort of 333 patients by Pei et al in China, renal failure developed in only 5% of cases. (663). This difference is explained by the prolonged duration of symptoms prior to consultation in our study.

In our series of 364 patients, we found that
7.6% thromboembolic complications. In a Dutch cohort involving 184 patients hospitalized in intensive care, the cumulative probability of venous thromboembolism (VTE), without systematic screening but with thromboprophylaxis, was 27% at around 2 weeks' follow-up. Moreover, PE was the most frequent complication (25.8%). A prospective French cohort, conducted in several intensive care units, reported a VTE rate of 17% despite systematic thromboprophylaxis (664). Helms et al found an 18% incidence

of thromboembolic complications in a population of 150 intensive care patients (665).

With regard to infectious complications (45, 666)the rate of nosocomial infections in patients with COVID-19 varies from study to study, ranging from 0.6% to 45%. Nosocomial infections can be bacterial, viral or fungal in origin. During hospitalization, bacterial infection can occur in 14% of cases, and seems to be part of a nosocomial context involving infections with multi-resistant bacteria in series where the percentage of patients on antibiotics is very high. In the study by Zhou et al involving 191 patients, 95% received antibiotics, whereas a well-defined bacterial complication was proven in only 28 (15%) patients (667).

Of 99 patients with COVID-19 described in the study by Chen et al, 4 (4%) had nosocomial fungal infections, including C. albicans and C. glabrata (668). Cases of pulmonary aspergillosis have also been reported (69). In our study, no cases of fungal infection were found.

In our series, dysthyroidism associated with COVID-19 infection was 32.4%. In the literature, this frequency ranges from 1.2% to 61.9%.

A meta-analysis published in October 2022, showed that the prevalence of thyroid dysfunction among 9707 COVID-19 patients was 15% (21). In an Indian study by Dutta et al, including 236 patients, dysthyroidism was reported in 33.9% of cases presenting with SARS-CoV-2 pneumopathy (70). Khoo et al. (71)Lui et al. (72) and Siso- almiral et al. (73) reported prevalence rates of 13.5%, 7.4% and 4.4% respectively.

As for comorbidities, our study revealed no difference between the two groups. Nevertheless, in a prospective study (74) carried out in one of Hong Kong's hospitals among patients diagnosed as seropositive for COVID-19 between July 21, 2020 and May 20, 2021, it was found that patients who developed thyroid balance disturbance were older and had more comorbidities, particularly diabetes.

During the acute phase, patients with dysthyroidism had worse biological profiles: higher levels of leukocytes, pro-inflammatory factors (higher CRP) and lower haematological parameters (including lymphocyte and platelet counts). (74,775). This is consistent with our study. Certainly, it is difficult to explain the relationship between platelet count and the onset of thyroid disorder. However, numerous studies in the COVID-19 population have revealed that thrombocytopenia may be a marker of inflammation and an adverse prognostic factor (76).

Studies have shown that patients with low TSH have a higher temperature (77) and a poorer prognosis (60)which is not consistent with our survey.

In our study, patients with dysthyroidism had a more severe clinical picture; SAPS II score, use of VMI, occurrence of septic EDC and use of vasoactive drugs were significantly higher. An Indian study (78)involving 100 patients with COVID-19 hospitalized in the intensive care unit, found that those who developed a disturbed thyroid balance had a significantly higher APACHE II score. Moreover, according to the study by Zou et al. (79)an association was reported between thyroid balance disturbance and the severity of the clinical picture (extension of pulmonary involvement ≥50% within 24H or 48H, use of IMV, occurrence of EDC). This could be explained by the fact that thyroid hormones can affect muscle strength (80). Indeed, during hypothyroidism, reversible respiratory muscle weakness and diaphragmatic dysfunction have been observed (81). Hence, patients who developed dysthyroidism were significantly more likely to require OHD or VMI. Also, a meta-analysis (82) found that patients in the "Dysthyroidism" group presented a more severe clinical picture (hemodynamic instability) and left ventricular ejection fraction was significantly lower (52 ± 10% vs. 56 ± 8%; $p<0.001$). These results were explained by the fact that thyroid hormones, particularly T3, are involved in myocardial contraction.

In our study, comparing the two groups, extension of lung lesions on CT was not significant, yet parenchymal involvement ≥ 50% was significantly associated with mortality.

In the study by Swistek et al, dysthyroidism was associated with mortality in COVID-19-positive patients with lung involvement of 50% or less. Kaplan-Meier curves indicated a lower probability of survival in patients with thyroid balance disturbance when CT parenchymal involvement was 50% or less. No significant difference was found for parenchymal involvement of more than 50%. (75).

Certainly, in the literature, the relationship between the occurrence of septic shock and dysthyroidism has been the subject of much discussion. The incidence of thyroid dysfunction was higher in hospitalized patients with septic shock, which corresponds to our study. This phenomenon is explained by numerous pathophysiological factors, including damage to the corticotropic axis, cytokine storm and damage to the thyrotropic axis (83, 884).

ARF has been reported in the literature as a prognostic factor in patients with COVID-19. This complication has also been shown to be a factor associated with dysthyroidism (85,86). Our series did not confirm these results. Indeed, the occurrence of AKI was comparable between the two groups.

In our study population, length of hospital stay was comparable between the two groups. These results contradicted a Polish study (75) which showed that patients with thyroid dysfunction had a significantly longer hospital stay than those who were healthy (10.5 IQR days [8-13] for the "Dysthyroidism" group versus 9.5 IQR days [7-12] for the "Euthyroidism" group; p=0 .003). Similarly, it has been shown that COVID-19 patients with thyroid balance disturbance are more likely to be hospitalized for more than

28 days (87). However, no such difference was found in a similar study (79,888).

Our study showed that dysthyroidism was a predictive factor for mortality in COVID-19 patients. These results are confirmed by the literature, which defines the various thyroid balance disturbances as a poor prognostic factor (89,90)Indeed, the occurrence of dysthyroidism was associated with disease severity. Its prevalence was 6.2% in mild to moderate forms versus 20.8% in severe forms, with a statistically significant difference (64).

Therapeutic management was always a controversial and nebulous subject in the context of COVID-19, insofar as it was still difficult to determine whether the disturbance in thyroid balance was a pathological condition or a means of adaptation by the organism (reduction in basic metabolic requirements in the event of acute aggression). (91, 992).

In the literature, published clinical studies aimed at assessing the effect of correction of thyroid disturbance in intensive care patients presented different modalities and divergent results. Two separate studies by Brent GA(93) and Acker CG et al (94)which applied different therapeutic protocols, no significant beneficial effect on mortality was observed in patients receiving substitution therapy. In fact, in the series by Acker et al. there was even an increase in mortality in patients with acute renal failure after T4 administration (94).

According to the French Society of Endocrinology, dysthyroidism associated with COVID-19 infection in the intensive care setting has been described as transient and spontaneously resolving in the majority of cases; the thyroid balance will normalize after recovery. In our study, we confirmed the diagnosis and adjusted management without systematic recourse to antithyroid drugs or hormone replacement. However, it was important not to overlook the presence of thyrotoxicosis, and to reinforce prevention of thromboembolic complications in these patients In addition, it was necessary to carry out a thyroid check-up at a distance.

In the multivariate study, dexamethasone corticosteroid therapy was found to be a preventive factor. Glucocorticoids interfere with thyroid hormone metabolism, and this can be explained by the blockage of peripheral T4 conversion with impaired TSH secretion, the fact that circulating thyroxine levels may affect cortisol transport and bioavailability (95).

In the multivariate study, preventive anticoagulation was also found to be a factor independently associated with dysthyroidism. Coagulopathy was the result of both systemic inflammation and a SARS-CoV-2-specific mechanism via ACE2 inhibition or endothelial injury. In addition to the anticoagulant effect, fractionated and unfractionated heparin displace thyroid hormone binding proteins, consequently affecting fT4 and fT3 measurements (95).

However, it should be pointed out that our study has a number of limitations. As the laboratory at Tahar Sfar Hospital in Mahdia only measures FT4 and TSH hormones, we were limited by technical problems in measuring FT3. As a result, we were unable to detect the occurrence of "low T3 syndrome". Once these tests have been requested, they are only carried out on admission. This prevents us from observing dynamic alterations in thyroid function over the course of the disease. Therefore, repeated thyroid hormone measurements at regular intervals would increase the validity of these results.

It has also been impossible to prevent certain factors from interfering with thyroid function, notably glucocorticoids and heparin. As a result, it is sometimes difficult to interpret thyroid function and differentiate dysthyroidism associated with COVID-19 infection from primary thyroid disorders.

Our study showed an association between thyroid balance disturbance and the severity of COVID-19. Indeed, further studies are needed to understand the prognostic significance of thyroid dysfunction in severe cases of COVID-19 and to investigate therapeutic approaches to reduce the poor outcomes associated with this clinical condition.

Finally, the literature reveals cases of post-viral subacute thyroiditis. Hence the need to be vigilant in cases of non-specific symptoms sometimes referred to as "post-disease syndrome", and to question the need for a thyroid work-up. A larger, longer-term study could complement these investigations.

CONCLUSION

The COVID-19 viral pandemic has disrupted global health and caused enormous morbidity and mortality. The disease, which first appeared in China in late 2019, has infected over 700 million people worldwide, causing more than 6 million deaths.

The main target of SARS-CoV-2 is invariably the lung, causing pneumonia of varying severity. Nevertheless, the range of associated diseases is very broad. Clinical manifestations range from pauci-symptomatic infection to severe pneumonia requiring oxygen therapy, even to a critical form requiring transfer to intensive care due to ARDS, and the cytokine storm has sometimes caused multiple visceral failures.

Thyroid dysfunction in patients with SARS-COV2 pneumonia was an increasingly common entity in intensive care units. However, its incidence and impact on mortality in COVID-19-positive patients were poorly studied in the literature.

We therefore carried out a single-center prospective study including 364 patients admitted to the intensive care unit of Tahar Sfar Hospital in Mahdia for treatment of SARS COV2 pneumonia during the period from September 2020 to September 2022.

The aim of our work was to determine the incidence of dysthyroidism associated with COVID-19 infection and its prognostic impact.

The median age of our patients was 61 years IQR [51-68]. The majority (34.9%) were in the 60-69 age bracket. They were predominantly male, with a sex ratio of 1.32. Hypertension (39.6%), followed by diabetes (35.4%) were the most frequent comorbidities.

The incidence of dysthyroidism in our study was 32.4%. Hyperthyroidism was found in 105 cases (89%), while hypothyroidism was detected in 13 cases (11%).

Mortality was 42.3%. The two major causes of death were refractory hypoxemia (53.9%) and refractory shock (34.9%).

Univariate analysis revealed that the group of patients with dysthyroidism was more severe: the SAPS II score was significantly higher. Similarly, use of mechanical ventilation, administration of catecholamines, rate of nosocomial infections and occurrence of septic DCI were significantly higher. Mortality was higher in the "Dysthyroidism" group (53.4% vs. 36.7%).

In the multivariate analysis, corticosteroid therapy and preventive anticoagulation were factors independently associated with dysthyroidism.

Larger-scale multicenter studies are needed to confirm these findings. Furthermore, to investigate the correlation between abnormal hormone dynamics and mortality during COVID-19, T3, T4 and TSH hormone dynamics need to be monitored at different time intervals.

BIBLIOGRAPHY

1 Bayarri VM, Sancho S, Campos C, Faus R, Simón JM, Porcar E, et al [The euthyroid sick syndrome in severe acute illness]. Presse Medicale Paris Fr 1983. Nov 2007;36(11 Pt 1):1550-6.

2. Peeters RP. Non thyroidal illness: to treat or not to treat? Ann Endocrinol. Sept 2007;68(4):224-8.

3 Lu H, Stratton CW, Tang YW. Outbreak of pneumonia of unknown etiology in Wuhan, China: The mystery and the miracle. J Med Virol. Apr 2020;92(4):401-2.

4. Sohrabi C, Alsafi Z, O'Neill N, Khan M, Kerwan A, Al-Jabir A, et al. World Health Organization declares global emergency: A review of the 2019 novel coronavirus (COVID-19). Int J Surg Lond Engl. Apr 2020;76:71-6.

5. Wu Z, McGoogan JM. Characteristics of and Important Lessons From the Coronavirus Disease 2019 (COVID-19) Outbreak in China: Summary of a Report of 72,314 Cases From the Chinese Center for Disease Control and Prevention. JAMA. Apr 7, 2020;323(13):1239-42.

6. Ding Y, He L, Zhang Q, Huang Z, Che X, Hou J, et al. Organ distribution of severe acute respiratory syndrome (SARS) associated coronavirus (SARS-CoV) in SARS patients: implications for pathogenesis and virus transmission pathways. J Pathol. June 2004;203(2):622-30.

7. Croce L, Gangemi D, Ancona G, Liboà F, Bendotti G, Minelli L, et al. The cytokine storm and thyroid hormone changes in COVID-19. J Endocrinol Invest. May 2021;44(5):891-904.

8. Takahashi T, Ellingson MK, Wong P, Israelow B, Lucas C, Klein J, et al. Sex differences in immune responses that underlie COVID-19 disease outcomes. Nature. Dec 2020;588(7837):315-20.

9 Knaus WA, Draper EA, Wagner DP, Zimmerman JE. APACHE II: a severity of disease classification system. Crit Care Med. Oct 1985;13(10):818-29.

10. Le Gall JR, Lemeshow S, Saulnier F. A new Simplified Acute Physiology Score (SAPS II) based on a European/North American multicenter study. JAMA. Dec 22 1993;270(24):2957-63.

11. Aissaoui O, El-bouz M, Bousfiha AA, Gueddari W, Chlilek A. Sepsis in children: protocol for rapid referral to pediatric resuscitation. Pan Afr Med J. 8 Jul 2021;39:189.

12. Thompson B, Moss M. A New Definition for the Acute Respiratory Distress Syndrome. Semin Respir Crit Care Med. August 11, 2013;34(04):441-7.

13. Khwaja A. KDIGO Clinical Practice Guidelines for Acute Kidney Injury. Nephron Clin Pract. August 7, 2012;120(4):c179-84.

14. Mahsouli A, Grillo M, Amini N, Acid S, Coche E, Ghaye B. Thoracic imaging of COVID-19. Louvain Med 2020 May-June; 139 (05-06): 360-367

15. Lodé B, Jalaber C, Orcel T, Morcet-Delattre T, Crespin N, Voisin S, et al. Imaging of COVID-19 pneumonia. J Imag Diagn Interv. Sept 2020;3(4):249-58.

16. Tang X, Du RH, Wang R, Cao TZ, Guan LL, Yang CQ, et al. Comparison of Hospitalized Patients With ARDS Caused by COVID-19 and H1N1. Chest. July 2020;158(1):195-205.

17. Gorini F, Bianchi F, Iervasi G. COVID-19 and Thyroid: Progress and Prospects.

Int J Environ Res Public Health. Sep 11, 2020;17(18):6630.

18. Lam SD, Bordin N, Waman VP, Scholes HM, Ashford P, Sen N, et al. SARS-CoV-2 spike protein predicted to form complexes with host receptor protein orthologues from a broad range of mammals. Sci Rep. 5 Oct 2020;10(1):16471.

19. Rotondi M, Coperchini F, Ricci G, Denegri M, Croce L, Ngnitejeu ST, et al. Detection of SARS-COV-2 receptor ACE-2 mRNA in thyroid cells: a clue for COVID-19-related subacute thyroiditis. J Endocrinol Invest. May 2021;44(5):1085-90.

20. Lisco G, De Tullio A, Jirillo E, Giagulli VA, De Pergola G, Guastamacchia E, et al. Thyroid and COVID-19: a review on pathophysiological, clinical and organizational aspects. J Endocrinol Invest. March 25, 2021;44(9):1801-14.

21. Mukhtar N, Bakhsh A, Alreshidi N, Aljomaiah A, Aljamei H, Alsudani N, et al. COVID-19 infection and thyroid function. Endocr Metab Sci. June 2022;7-8:100122.

22 Rossetti CL, Cazarin J, Hecht F, Beltrão FE de L, Ferreira ACF, Fortunato RS, et al. COVID-19 and thyroid function: What do we know so far? Front Endocrinol. 2022;13:1041676.

23. Caironi V, Pitoia F, Trimboli P. Thyroid Inconveniences With Vaccination Against SARS-CoV-2: The Size of the Matter. A Systematic Review. Front Endocrinol. 2022;13:900964.

24. Ippolito S, Gallo D, Rossini A, Patera B, Lanzo N, Fazzino GFM, et al. SARS-CoV-2 vaccine-associated subacute thyroiditis: insights from a systematic review. J Endocrinol Invest. June 2022;45(6):1189-200.

25. Vera-Lastra O, Ordinola Navarro A, Cruz Domiguez MP, Medina G, Sánchez Valadez TI, Jara LJ. Two Cases of Graves' Disease Following SARS-CoV-2 Vaccination: An Autoimmune/Inflammatory Syndrome Induced by Adjuvants. Thyroid Off J Am Thyroid Assoc. Sept 2021;31(9):1436-9.

26. Vojdani A, Kharrazian D. Potential antigenic cross-reactivity between SARS-CoV-2 and human tissue with a possible link to an increase in autoimmune diseases. Clin Immunol Orlando Fla. August 2020;217:108480.

27. Oliveira E, Parikh A, Lopez-Ruiz A, Carrilo M, Goldberg J, Cearras M, et al. ICU outcomes and survival in patients with severe COVID-19 in the largest health care system in central Florida. PloS One. 2021;16(3):e0249038.

28. Grasselli G, Greco M, Zanella A, Albano G, Antonelli M, Bellani G, et al. Risk Factors Associated With Mortality Among Patients With COVID-19 in Intensive Care Units in Lombardy, Italy. JAMA Intern Med. 1 Oct 2020;180(10):1345-55.

29. Yu Y, Xu D, Fu S, Zhang J, Yang X, Xu L, et al. Patients with COVID-19 in 19 ICUs in Wuhan, China: a cross-sectional study. Crit Care Lond Engl. May 14, 2020;24(1):219.

30. Elmadkouri H. Covid-19 at the Avicenne Military Hospital in Marrakech, Morocco: virological, epidemiological, clinical and evolutionary bases [doctoral thesis]. Marrakech Faculty of Medicine and Pharmacy; 2021.

31. Al Mutair A, Al Mutairi A, Zaidi ARZ, Salih S, Alhumaid S, Rabaan AA, et al. Clinical Predictors of COVID-19 Mortality Among Patients in Intensive Care Units: A Retrospective Study. Int J Gen Med. 2021;14:3719-28.

32 Foresta C, Rocca MS, Di Nisio A. Gender susceptibility to COVID-19: a review of the putative role of sex hormones and X chromosome. J Endocrinol Invest. 2021;44(5):951-6.

33. Donamou J, Bangoura A, Camara LM, Camara D, Traoré DA, Abékan RJM, et al. Epidemiological and clinical characteristics of COVID-19 patients admitted to intensive care at Donka Hospital in Conakry, Guinea: descriptive study of the first 140 hospitalized cases. Anesth Réanimation. March 2021;7(2):102-9.

34. Singh AK, Gupta R, Ghosh A, Misra A. Diabetes in COVID-19: Prevalence, pathophysiology, prognosis and practical considerations. Diabetes Metab Syndr. 2020;14(4):303-10.

35 Desvaux É, Faucher JF. Covid-19: clinical aspects and main elements of management. Rev Francoph Lab. Nov 2020;2020(526):40-7.

36 Hariyanto H, Yahya CQ, Aritonang RCA. Severe COVID-19 in the intensive care unit: a case series. J Med Case Reports. May 3, 2021;15(1):259.

37. Xu Y, Xu Z, Liu X, Cai L, Zheng H, Huang Y, et al. Clinical Findings of COVID-19 Patients Admitted to Intensive Care Units in Guangdong Province, China: A Multicenter, Retrospective, Observational Study. Front Med. 2020;7:576457.

38. SAHA A, AHSAN MM, QUADER TU, SHOHAN MUS, NAHER S, DUTTA P, et al. Characteristics, management and outcomes of critically ill COVID-19 patients admitted to ICU in hospitals in Bangladesh: a retrospective study. J Prev Med Hyg. 29 Apr 2021;62(1):E33-45.

39. Monk M, Torres J, Vickery K, Jayaraman G, Sarva ST, Kesavan R. A Comparison of ICU Mortality Scoring Systems Applied to COVID-19. Cureus. 15(2):e35423

40. Raschke RA, Agarwal S, Rangan P, Heise CW, Curry SC. Discriminant Accuracy of the SOFA Score for Determining the Probable Mortality of Patients With COVID-19 Pneumonia Requiring Mechanical Ventilation. JAMA. Apr 13, 2021;325(14):1469-70.

41. Xu J, Yang X, Yang L, Zou X, Wang Y, Wu Y, et al. Clinical course and predictors of 60-day mortality in 239 critically ill patients with COVID-19: a multicenter retrospective study from Wuhan, China. Crit Care Lond Engl. 6 Jul 2020;24(1):394.

42. Mitra AR, Fergusson NA, Lloyd-Smith E, Wormsbecker A, Foster D, Karpov A, et al. Baseline characteristics and outcomes of patients with COVID-19 admitted to intensive care units in Vancouver, Canada: a case series. CMAJ Can Med Assoc J J Assoc Medicale Can. June 29, 2020;192(26):E694-701.

43 COVID-ICU Group on behalf of the REVA Network and the COVID-ICU Investigators. Clinical characteristics and day-90 outcomes of 4244 critically ill adults with COVID-19: a prospective cohort study. Intensive Care Med. Jan 2021;47(1):60-73.

44. Lodé B, Jalaber C, Orcel T, Morcet-Delattre T, Crespin N, Voisin S, et al. Imaging of COVID-19 pneumonia. J Imag Diagn Interv. Sept 2020;3(4):249.

45. Report on updating the management of patients with Covid-19. Haut Conseil de la santé publique. July 2020

46. Verity R, Okell LC, Dorigatti I, Winskill P, Whittaker C, Imai N, et al. Estimates of the severity of coronavirus disease 2019: a model-based analysis. Lancet Infect Dis. June 2020;20(6):669-77.

47. Xu J, Yang X, Yang L, Zou X, Wang Y, Wu Y, et al. Clinical course and predictors of 60-day mortality in 239 critically ill patients with COVID-19: a multicenter retrospective study from Wuhan, China. Crit Care Lond Engl. 6 Jul 2020;24(1):394.

48 Zhang C, Shi L, Wang FS. Liver injury in COVID-19: management and challenges. Lancet Gastroenterol Hepatol. May 2020;5(5):428-30.

49. Ayanian S, Reyes J, Lynn L, Teufel K. The association between biomarkers and clinical outcomes in novel coronavirus pneumonia in a US cohort. Biomark Med. August 2020;14(12):1091-7.

50. Guan W jie, Ni Z yi, Hu Y, Liang W hua, Ou C quan, He J xing, et al. Clinical Characteristics of Coronavirus Disease 2019 in China. N Engl J Med. Apr 30, 2020;382(18):1708-20.

51. Zhou F, Yu T, Du R, Fan G, Liu Y, Liu Z, et al. Clinical course and risk factors for mortality of adult inpatients with COVID-19 in Wuhan, China: a retrospective cohort study. Lancet Lond Engl. March 28, 2020;395(10229):1054-62.

52. African COVID-19 Critical Care Outcomes Study (ACCCOS) Investigators. Patient care and clinical outcomes for patients with COVID-19 infection admitted to African high-care or intensive care units (ACCCOS): a multicentre, prospective, observational cohort study. Lancet Lond Engl. May 22, 2021;397(10288):1885-94.

53. RECOVERY Collaborative Group, Horby P, Lim WS, Emberson JR, Mafham M, Bell JL, et al. Dexamethasone in Hospitalized Patients with Covid-19. N Engl J Med. Feb 25, 2021;384(8):693-704.

54. Ramakrishnan S, Nicolau DV, Langford B, Mahdi M, Jeffers H, Mwasuku C, et al. Inhaled budesonide in the treatment of early COVID-19 (STOIC): a phase 2, open-label, randomised controlled trial. Lancet Respir Med. Jul 2021;9(7):763-72.

55. Yu LM, Bafadhel M, Dorward J, Hayward G, Saville BR, Gbinigie O, et al. Inhaled budesonide for COVID-19 in people at high risk of complications in the community in the UK (PRINCIPLE): a randomised, controlled, open-label, adaptive platform trial. The Lancet. Sept 2021;398(10303):843-55.

56. Chifu I, Detomas M, Dischinger U, Kimpel O, Megerle F, Hahner S, et al. Management of Patients With Glucocorticoid-Related Diseases and COVID-19. Front Endocrinol. 2021;12:705214.

57. Alexaki VI, Henneicke H. The Role of Glucocorticoids in the Management of COVID-19. Horm Metab Res Horm Stoffwechselforschung Horm Metab. janv 2021;53(1):9-15.

58. Abdessamad DAOUI, Profil épidémiologique, clinique et biologique des patients COVID-19 hospitalisés au CHR Hassan II d'Agadir, July 2021.

59. Mousavi S, Moradi M, Khorshidahmad T, Motamedi M. Anti-Inflammatory Effects of Heparin and Its Derivatives: A Systematic Review. Adv Pharmacol Sci. 2015;2015:507151.

60. Matera MG, Rogliani P, Calzetta L, Cazzola M. Pharmacological management of COVID-19 patients with ARDS (CARDS): A narrative review. Respir Med. Sept 2020;171:106114.

61. Tazi Mezalek Z. COVID-19: coagulopathy and thrombosis. Rev Med Interne. Feb 2021;42(2):93-100.

62. Hospital course of Covid-19 patients during the first wave of the epidemic. Les dossiers de la DREES n° 67.October 2020

63. Hirsch JS, Ng JH, Ross DW, Sharma P, Shah HH, Barnett RL, et al. Acute kidney injury in patients hospitalized with COVID-19. Kidney Int. Jul 2020;98(1):209-18.

64. Pei G, Zhang Z, Peng J, Liu L, Zhang C, Yu C, et al. Renal Involvement and Early Prognosis in Patients with COVID-19 Pneumonia. J Am Soc Nephrol JASN. June 2020;31(6):1157-65.

65. Casini A, Fontana P, Glauser F, Robert-Ebadi H, Righini M, Blondon M. Venous thrombotic risk induced by SARS-CoV-2: prevalence, recommendations and outlook. Rev Médicale Suisse. 2020;16(692):951-4.

66. Lai CC, Wang CY, Hsueh PR. Co-infections among patients with COVID-19: The need for combination therapy with non-anti-SARS-CoV-2 agents? J Microbiol Immunol Infect. August 2020;53(4):505-12.

67. Zhou F, Yu T, Du R, Fan G, Liu Y, Liu Z, et al. Clinical course and risk factors for mortality of adult inpatients with COVID-19 in Wuhan, China: a retrospective cohort study. Lancet Lond Engl. March 28, 2020;395(10229):1054-62.

68. Chen N, Zhou M, Dong X, Qu J, Gong F, Han Y, et al. Epidemiological and clinical characteristics of 99 cases of 2019 novel coronavirus pneumonia in Wuhan, China: a descriptive study. Lancet Lond Engl. Feb 15, 2020;395(10223):507-13.

69. Lescure FX, Bouadma L, Nguyen D, Parisey M, Wicky PH, Behillil S, et al. Clinical and virological data of the first cases of COVID-19 in Europe: a case series. Lancet Infect Dis. June 2020;20(6):697-706.

70. Dutta A, Jevalikar G, Sharma R, Farooqui KJ, Mahendru S, Dewan A, et al. Low FT3 is an independent marker of disease severity in patients hospitalized for COVID-19. Endocr Connect. 11 Nov 2021;10(11):1455.

71. Khoo B, Tan T, Clarke SA, Mills EG, Patel B, Modi M, et al. Thyroid Function Before, During, and After COVID-19. J Clin Endocrinol Metab. Jan 23, 2021;106(2):e803-11.

72. Lui DTW, Lee CH, Chow WS, Lee ACH, Tam AR, Fong CHY, et al. Thyroid Dysfunction in Relation to Immune Profile, Disease Status, and Outcome in 191 Patients with COVID-19. J Clin Endocrinol Metab. Jan 23, 2021;106(2):e926-35.

73. Sisó-Almirall A, Kostov B, Mas-Heredia M, Vilanova-Rotllan S, Sequeira-Aymar E, Sans-Corrales M, et al. Prognostic factors in Spanish COVID-19 patients: A case series from Barcelona. PLoS ONE. August 21, 2020;15(8):e0237960.

74. Lui DTW, Lee CH, Chow WS, Lee ACH, Tam AR, Cheung CYY, et al. Development of a prediction score (ThyroCOVID) for identifying abnormal thyroid function in COVID-19 patients. J Endocrinol Invest. 13 Jul 2022;45(11):2149-56.

75 .Świstek M, Broncel M, Gorzelak-Pabiś P, Morawski P, Fabiś M, Woźniak E. Euthyroid Sick Syndrome as a Prognostic Indicator of COVID-19 Pulmonary Involvement, Associated With Poorer Disease Prognosis and Increased Mortality. Endocr Pract Off J Am Coll Endocrinol Am Assoc Clin Endocrinol. May 2022;28(5):494-501.

76. Yang X, Yang Q, Wang Y, Wu Y, Xu J, Yu Y, et al. Thrombocytopenia and its association with mortality in patients with COVID-19. J Thromb Haemost JTH. June 2020;18(6):1469-72.

77. Lui DTW, Fung MMH, Chiu KWH, Lee CH, Chow WS, Lee ACH, et al. Higher SARS-CoV-2 viral loads correlated with smaller thyroid volumes on ultrasound among male COVID-19 survivors. Endocrine. 2021;74(2):205-14.

78. Mahashabde M, Murukoti SR, Chaudhary G, Kanchi G, Patil R. Study of Thyroid Functions in critically ill Patients admitted in Medical Intensive Care Unit and its Correlation with Critical Care Scoring Acute Physiology and Chronic Health Evaluation III. J Assoc Physicians India. Jul 2022;70(7):11-2.

79. Zou R, Wu C, Zhang S, Wang G, Zhang Q, Yu B, et al. Euthyroid Sick Syndrome in Patients With COVID-19. Front Endocrinol. 2020;11:566439.

80. Boelen A, Kwakkel J, Fliers E. Beyond low plasma T3: local thyroid hormone metabolism during inflammation and infection. Endocr Rev. Oct 2011;32(5):670-93.

81. Siafakas NM, Salesiotou V, Filaditaki V, Tzanakis N, Thalassinos N, Bouros D. Respiratory muscle strength in hypothyroidism. Chest. July 1992;102(1):189-94.

82. Chang CY, Chien YJ, Lin PC, Chen CS, Wu MY. Nonthyroidal Illness Syndrome and Hypothyroidism in Ischemic Heart Disease Population: A Systematic Review and Meta-Analysis. J Clin Endocrinol Metab. August 1, 2020;105(8):dgaa310.

83. Mönig H, Arendt T, Meyer M, Kloehn S, Bewig B. Activation of the hypothalamo-pituitary-adrenal axis in response to septic or non-septic diseases--implications for the euthyroid sick syndrome. Intensive Care Med. Dec 1999;25(12):1402-6.

84. Castro I, Quisenberry L, Calvo RM, Obregon MJ, Lado-Abeal J. Septic shock non-thyroidal illness syndrome causes hypothyroidism and conditions for reduced sensitivity to thyroid hormone. J Mol Endocrinol. Apr 2013;50(2):255-66.

85. Ertuğlu LA, Kanbay A, Afşar B, Elsürer Afşar R, Kanbay M. COVID-19 and acute kidney injury. Tuberk Ve Toraks. dec 2020;68(4):407-18.

86. Tognini S, Marchini F, Dardano A, Polini A, Ferdeghini M, Castiglioni M, et al. Non-thyroidal illness syndrome and short-term survival in a hospitalized older population. Age Ageing. Jan 2010;39(1):46-50.

87. Zhang Y, Lin F, Tu W, Zhang J, Choudhry AA, Ahmed O, et al. Thyroid dysfunction may be associated with poor outcomes in patients with COVID-19. Mol Cell Endocrinol. 5 Feb 2021;521:111097.

88. Schwarz Y, Percik R, Oberman B, Yaffe D, Zimlichman E, Tirosh A. Sick Euthyroid Syndrome on Presentation of Patients With COVID-19: A Potential Marker for Disease Severity. Endocr Pract. Feb 2021;27(2):101-9.

89. Croce L, Gangemi D, Ancona G, Liboà F, Bendotti G, Minelli L, et al. The cytokine storm and thyroid hormone changes in COVID-19. J Endocrinol Invest. May 2021;44(5):891-904.

90. Lui DTW, Lee CH, Chow WS, Lee ACH, Tam AR, Fong CHY, et al. Role of non-thyroidal illness syndrome in predicting adverse outcomes in COVID-19 patients predominantly of mild-to-moderate severity. Clin Endocrinol (Oxf). Sept 2021;95(3):469-77.

91. Warner MH, Beckett GJ. Mechanisms behind the non-thyroidal illness syndrome: an update. J Endocrinol. Apr 1, 2010;205(1):1-13.

92. Lechan RM. The dilemma of the Nonthyroidal Illness Syndrome. Acta Bio-Medica Atenei Parm. Dec 2008;79(3):165-71.

93. Brent GA, Hershman JM. Thyroxine Therapy in Patients with Severe Nonthyroidal Illnesses and Low Serum Thyroxine Concentration*. J Clin Endocrinol Metab. July 1986;63(1):1-8.

94. Acker CG, Singh AR, Flick RP, Bernardini J, Greenberg A, Johnson JP. A trial of thyroxine in acute renal failure. Kidney Int. 1 Jan 2000;57(1):293-8.

95. Tian Y, Zhao J, Wang T, Wang H, Yao J, Wang S, et al. Thyroid diseases are associated with coronavirus disease 2019 infection. Front Endocrinol. Sep 2, 2022;13:952049.

APPENDIX

Appendix I: Reference values used to interpret biological results

Balance sheet	Reference value
Hyperleukocytosis (elements/mm^3)	>11000
Leukopenia (elements/mm^3)	<4000
Lymphopenia (elements/mm^3)	<1500
Thrombocytopenia (elements/mm^3)	< 150 (10*3/mm3)
Thrombocytosis (elements/mm^3)	>400 (10*3/mm3)
TP decreased (%) (elements/mm^3)	<70
High CRP (mg/L)	<6
Hyper-uremia (mmol/L)	>7.5
Hyper-creatinemia (µmol/L)	Age-related clearance
AST (UI/l)	Between 8 - 30: men Between 6 and 25: women
ALAT (IU/l)	Between 8 and 30: men Between 6 and 25: women.
Hypo-kalemia (mmol/L)	< 3.5
Hyperkalemia (mmol/L)	>5.5
Hypo-natremia (mmol/L)	< 135
Hyper-natremia (mmol/L)	>145
TSH (mIU/L)	0.3 - 5.6
FT4 (pmol/L)	7.8-14.8
Arterial blood pH	7.38-7.42
Oxygen saturation (sO2) (%)	95-100
Partial pressure of carbon dioxide (PCO2) (mm Hg)	38-42
partial pressure of oxygen (PaO2) (mm Hg)	80-100
Bicarbonate (HCO3) (mmol/l)	22-26
Lactates (mmol/l)	1-1.5

Summary

In addition to its respiratory tropism, covid-19 can cause systemic symptoms, including thyroid damage. The aim of our work was to study the incidence of thyroid dysfunction in patients with SARS-COV-2 pneumonia and its prognostic impact. It is a prospective study including patients admitted for covid-19 pneumonia between September 2020 and August 2022 and having a thyroid balance disturbance. We included 364 patients. The incidence of dysthyroidism was 32.4% (89% hyperthyroidism and 11% hypothyroidism). SAPS II score, use of mechanical ventilation, catecholamine administration, nosocomial infection rate, occurrence of septic DCI and mortality were significantly higher in the dysthyroidism group. In the multivariate analysis, corticosteroid therapy and preventive anticoagulation were factors independently associated with dysthyroidism. Larger, longer-term studies could complement this work.

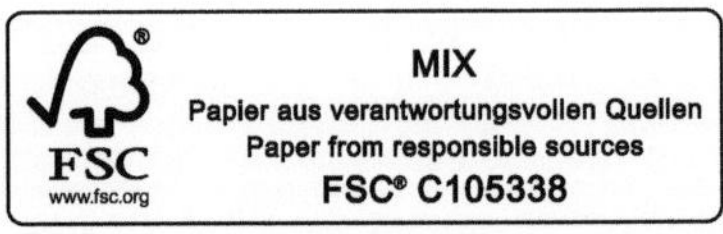

Printed by Books on Demand GmbH, Norderstedt / Germany